LOW RESIDUE DIET COOKBOOK

Deliciously Simple Recipes for a Gentle Digestion

T. JOHN

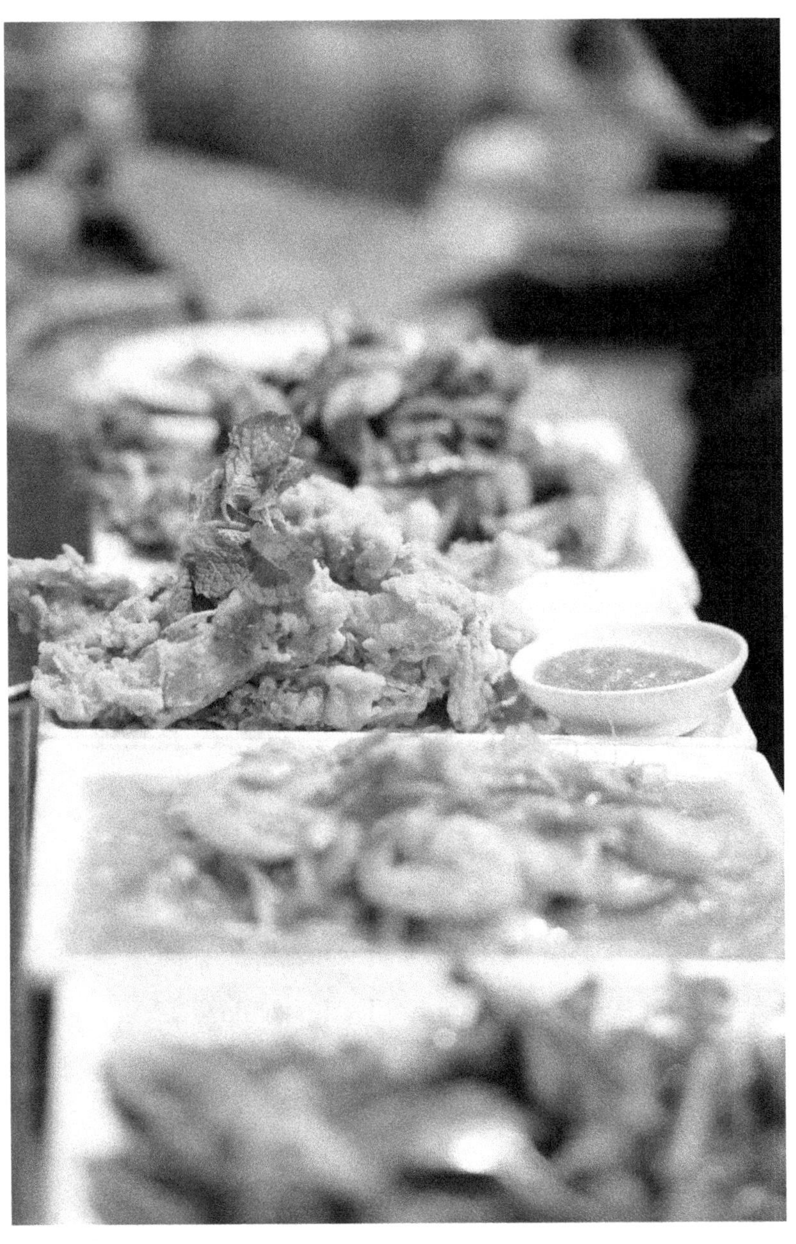

TABLE OF CONTENTS

Dinner Recipes 39

CONCLUSION 88

INTRODUCTION

W elcome to our Low Residue Diet Cookbook. In this introductory section, we will explore the fundamental concepts and principles behind the low residue diet. It is essential to have a clear understanding of this dietary approach before diving into the delicious recipes that lie ahead.

The low residue diet is a specialized eating plan designed to reduce the amount and frequency of bowel movements. It is commonly recommended for individuals who have undergone certain medical procedures, such as surgery or radiation therapy, or those who suffer from digestive disorders like Crohn's disease, ulcerative colitis, or diverticulitis. This diet aims to minimize the consumption of high-fiber foods, which can be difficult to digest and may irritate the gastrointestinal tract.

Benefits and Purpose of a Low Residue Diet

The primary purpose of following a low residue diet is to provide relief and promote healing for individuals with specific digestive conditions. By reducing the intake of bulky and high-fiber foods, the digestive system is given a chance to rest and recover. This can alleviate symptoms such as abdominal pain, diarrhea, and bloating.

Moreover, a low residue diet can help to manage inflammation and reduce the risk of complications in individuals with inflammatory bowel diseases. It allows the intestines to heal and prevents further damage to the gastrointestinal tract. Additionally, this dietary approach may also be recommended as a temporary measure before or after surgery to facilitate the healing process.

Guidelines and Considerations for a Low Residue Diet

Before embarking on a low residue diet, it is crucial to consult with a healthcare professional or a registered dietitian. They will be able to provide personalized guidance and tailor the diet to your specific needs. While the principles of a low residue diet remain consistent, individual variations may be necessary to ensure optimal nutrition and meet specific dietary requirements.

In general, a low residue diet involves avoiding or limiting certain types of foods. These include high-fiber grains, whole grains, seeds, nuts, raw fruits and vegetables, legumes, and tough meats. Instead, the diet emphasizes low-fiber alternatives and easily digestible foods such as refined grains, cooked fruits and vegetables without skins or seeds, lean proteins, and dairy products.

It is important to note that a low residue diet should not be followed for an extended period without medical supervision. The restriction of fiber can lead to a reduced intake of essential nutrients and may impact bowel regularity in the long term. Therefore, it is recommended to transition to a regular, well-balanced diet as soon as your healthcare provider deems it appropriate.

Navigating the Low Residue Diet Cookbook

Now that you have a solid understanding of the low residue diet and its benefits, you are ready to embark on your culinary journey through the rest of this cookbook. The subsequent chapters will guide you through a variety of delicious recipes specifically tailored to fit within the parameters of a low residue diet.

Each chapter focuses on a different meal category, including breakfast, lunch, dinner, snacks, appetizers, desserts, and smoothies. Within each category, you will find a selection of carefully curated recipes that are not only low in residue but also packed with flavor and nutrition. We have made sure to include a diverse range of options to cater to various dietary preferences and restrictions.

Throughout the cookbook, you will find helpful tips, substitution suggestions, and nutritional information accompanying each recipe. These additional details will empower you to make informed decisions about your dietary choices and ensure you are meeting your nutritional needs while enjoying a flavorful and satisfying culinary experience.

Breakfast Recipes

These breakfast recipes provide a variety of options to start your day with delicious and nourishing meals. Whether you prefer a warm bowl of oatmeal, a protein-packed frittata, or a refreshing yogurt parfait, these recipes will help you kick start your mornings on a satisfying note. Experiment with different flavors and ingredients to customize these breakfast recipes to your liking. Enjoy the most important meal of the day with these tasty and easy-to-make dishes.

Creamy Banana Oatmeal

Ingredients:

- 1 cup rolled oats
- 2 cups milk (dairy or plant-based)
- 1 ripe banana, mashed
- 1 tablespoon honey or maple syrup (optional)
- 1/2 teaspoon vanilla extract
- Pinch of salt
- Toppings: sliced banana, chopped nuts, cinnamon (optional)

Instructions:

1. In a saucepan, bring the milk to a gentle boil over medium heat.
2. Stir in the rolled oats and reduce the heat to low.
3. Add the mashed banana, honey or maple syrup (if using), vanilla extract, and salt. Mix well.
4. Cook the oats, stirring occasionally, for about 5-7 minutes or until they reach your desired consistency.
5. Remove the saucepan from the heat and let the oatmeal rest for a minute.
6. Serve the creamy banana oatmeal in bowls and garnish with sliced banana, chopped nuts, and a sprinkle of cinnamon, if desired.

Scrambled Eggs with Spinach and Feta

Ingredients:

- 4 large eggs
- 1 cup fresh spinach leaves
- 1/4 cup crumbled feta cheese
- Salt and pepper to taste
- 1 tablespoon olive oil or butter

Instructions:

1. In a bowl, beat the eggs until well combined. Season with salt and pepper.
2. Heat the olive oil or butter in a non-stick skillet over medium heat.
3. Add the spinach leaves to the skillet and sauté until wilted.
4. Pour the beaten eggs into the skillet and stir gently with a spatula.
5. Continue cooking the eggs, stirring occasionally, until they are almost set.
6. Sprinkle the crumbled feta cheese over the eggs and cook for another minute or until the cheese melts.
7. Remove the skillet from the heat and transfer the scrambled eggs with spinach and feta to a plate.
8. Serve hot with toast or your favorite breakfast sides.

Blueberry Yogurt Parfait

Ingredients:

- 1 cup Greek yogurt
- 1/2 cup fresh blueberries
- 1/4 cup granola

- 1 tablespoon honey (optional)
- Fresh mint leaves for garnish (optional)

Instructions:

1. In a glass or a bowl, layer half of the Greek yogurt.
2. Add half of the blueberries on top of the yogurt.
3. Sprinkle half of the granola over the blueberries.
4. Repeat the layers with the remaining yogurt, blueberries, and granola.
5. Drizzle honey on top, if desired.
6. Garnish with fresh mint leaves, if using.
7. Serve the blueberry yogurt parfait immediately or refrigerate for later enjoyment.

Vegetable Frittata

Ingredients:

- 6 large eggs
- 1/4 cup milk (dairy or plant-based)
- 1/2 cup diced bell peppers (any color)
- 1/2 cup diced zucchini
- 1/4 cup diced red onion
- 1/4 cup chopped cherry tomatoes

- 1/4 cup shredded cheddar cheese
- 1 tablespoon olive oil
- Salt and pepper to taste

Instructions:

1. Preheat the oven to 350°F (175°C).
2. In a bowl, whisk together the eggs, milk, salt, and pepper.
3. Heat the olive oil in an oven-safe skillet over medium heat.
4. Add the bell peppers, zucchini, and red onion to the skillet. Sauté for a few minutes until slightly softened.
5. Pour the egg mixture over the sautéed vegetables in the skillet.
6. Sprinkle the chopped cherry tomatoes and shredded cheddar cheese evenly over the eggs.
7. Cook the frittata on the stovetop for about 3-4 minutes or until the edges start to set.
8. Transfer the skillet to the preheated oven and bake for 15-20 minutes or until the eggs are fully set and the top is golden.

9. Remove the skillet from the oven and let the frittata cool for a few minutes.

10. Slice the vegetable frittata into wedges and serve warm.

Apple Cinnamon Pancakes

Ingredients:

- 1 cup all-purpose flour
- 2 tablespoons granulated sugar
- 2 teaspoons baking powder
- 1/2 teaspoon ground cinnamon
- 1/4 teaspoon salt
- 1 cup milk (dairy or plant-based)
- 1 large egg
- 2 tablespoons unsalted butter, melted
- 1 apple, peeled and finely chopped
- Maple syrup and sliced apples for serving

Instructions:

1. In a large bowl, whisk together the flour, sugar, baking powder, cinnamon, and salt.

2. In a separate bowl, whisk together the milk, egg, and melted butter.

3. Pour the wet ingredients into the dry ingredients and stir until just combined. Do not overmix.

4. Gently fold in the finely chopped apple.

5. Heat a non-stick skillet or griddle over medium heat and lightly grease it with butter or cooking spray.

6. Pour 1/4 cup of the pancake batter onto the skillet for each pancake.

7. Cook until bubbles form on the surface, then flip the pancake and cook for another minute or until golden brown.

8. Repeat with the remaining batter.

9. Serve the apple cinnamon pancakes warm with maple syrup and sliced apples on top.

Quinoa Breakfast Bowl

Ingredients:

- 1 cup cooked quinoa
- 1/2 cup Greek yogurt
- 1/4 cup fresh berries (such as strawberries, blueberries, or raspberries)

- 2 tablespoons chopped nuts (such as almonds or walnuts)
- 1 tablespoon honey or maple syrup (optional)
- A sprinkle of cinnamon (optional)

Instructions:

1. In a bowl, combine the cooked quinoa and Greek yogurt.
2. Top the quinoa and yogurt mixture with fresh berries and chopped nuts.
3. Drizzle honey or maple syrup on top, if desired.
4. Sprinkle a bit of cinnamon over the bowl, if using.
5. Mix all the ingredients together gently.
6. Enjoy the nutritious and delicious quinoa breakfast bowl.

Chia Seed Pudding with Berries

Ingredients:

- 1/4 cup chia seeds
- 1 cup milk (dairy or plant-based)
- 1 tablespoon honey or maple syrup
- 1/2 teaspoon vanilla extract

- 1/2 cup fresh berries (such as strawberries, blueberries, or raspberries)
- Optional toppings: chopped nuts, coconut flakes, or additional berries

Instructions:

1. In a bowl, whisk together the chia seeds, milk, honey or maple syrup, and vanilla extract.
2. Let the mixture sit for about 5 minutes, then whisk again to prevent clumping.
3. Cover the bowl and refrigerate overnight or for at least 2 hours to allow the chia seeds to absorb the liquid and form a pudding-like consistency.
4. Before serving, give the chia seed pudding a good stir.
5. Spoon the pudding into serving bowls or glasses.
6. Top with fresh berries and any other desired toppings, such as chopped nuts or coconut flakes.
7. Enjoy the creamy and nutritious chia seed pudding for breakfast.

Almond Butter Toast with Sliced Bananas

Ingredients:

- 2 slices of whole grain bread, toasted
- 2 tablespoons almond butter
- 1 banana, sliced
- Honey or a sprinkle of cinnamon (optional)

Instructions:

1. Spread almond butter evenly on each slice of toasted bread.
2. Arrange the sliced bananas on top of the almond butter.
3. Drizzle honey on top or sprinkle a bit of cinnamon, if desired.
4. Serve the almond butter toast with sliced bananas as a quick and satisfying breakfast option.

Baked Omelette Muffins

Ingredients:

- 6 large eggs
- 1/4 cup milk (dairy or plant-based)

- 1/2 cup diced vegetables (such as bell peppers, spinach, onions, or mushrooms)
- 1/4 cup shredded cheddar cheese
- Salt and pepper to taste
- Cooking spray or butter for greasing the muffin tin

Instructions:

1. Preheat the oven to 350°F (175°C) and lightly grease a muffin tin with cooking spray or butter.
2. In a bowl, whisk together the eggs, milk, salt, and pepper.
3. Stir in the diced vegetables and shredded cheddar cheese.
4. Pour the egg mixture evenly into the greased muffin tin, filling each cup about 3/4 full.
5. Bake for 15-20 minutes or until the omelette muffins are set and slightly golden on top.
6. Remove the muffin tin from the oven and let the omelette muffins cool for a few minutes.
7. Carefully remove the muffins from the tin and serve them warm or at room temperature.

Avocado and Tomato Breakfast Wrap

Ingredients:

- 1 large tortilla or wrap of your choice
- 1 ripe avocado, sliced
- 1 tomato, sliced
- 2-3 slices of cooked bacon or vegetarian bacon substitute (optional)
- Handful of fresh spinach leaves
- Salt and pepper to taste

Instructions:

1. Lay the tortilla or wrap flat on a clean surface.
2. Arrange the sliced avocado, tomato, bacon (if using), and spinach leaves on the tortilla.
3. Season with salt and pepper to taste.
4. Tightly roll up the tortilla, folding in the sides as you go.
5. Slice the avocado and tomato breakfast wrap in half or into smaller pieces for easier handling.
6. Enjoy this flavorful and nutritious wrap as a filling breakfast option.

Lunch Recipes

In this chapter, we will explore delicious and nutritious Lunch recipes that are perfect for those following a low residue diet. These recipes offer a variety of flavors and ingredients to keep your taste buds satisfied while still being gentle on your digestive system.

Chicken and Rice Soup

Ingredients:

- 1 tablespoon olive oil
- 1 onion, diced
- 2 carrots, peeled and sliced
- 2 celery stalks, sliced
- 2 cloves of garlic, minced
- 4 cups chicken broth
- 2 cups cooked chicken, shredded
- 1 cup cooked rice
- 1 teaspoon dried thyme
- Salt and pepper to taste
- Fresh parsley, chopped (for garnish)

Instructions:

1. In a large pot, heat the olive oil over medium heat. Add the onion, carrots, celery, and garlic. Sauté until the vegetables are tender.
2. Pour in the chicken broth and bring to a boil. Reduce the heat to low and simmer for about 15 minutes.
3. Add the cooked chicken, rice, dried thyme, salt, and pepper. Stir well and simmer for an additional 10 minutes.
4. Adjust the seasoning if needed. Serve hot, garnished with fresh parsley.

Grilled Salmon with Steamed Vegetables

Ingredients:

- 2 salmon fillets
- 1 tablespoon olive oil
- Salt and pepper to taste
- 2 cups mixed vegetables (such as broccoli, carrots, and snap peas)

Instructions:

1. Preheat the grill to medium heat.

2. Brush the salmon fillets with olive oil and season with salt and pepper.

3. Place the salmon on the grill and cook for about 4-5 minutes per side, or until the fish is cooked through and flakes easily with a fork.

4. While the salmon is cooking, steam the mixed vegetables until tender.

5. Serve the grilled salmon with steamed vegetables on the side. Season with additional salt and pepper if desired.

Quinoa Salad with Roasted Vegetables

Ingredients:

- 1 cup quinoa, cooked and cooled
- 1 red bell pepper, diced
- 1 zucchini, diced
- 1 yellow squash, diced
- 1 small red onion, sliced
- 2 tablespoons olive oil
- 1 teaspoon dried oregano

- Salt and pepper to taste
- 2 tablespoons lemon juice
- 2 tablespoons fresh parsley, chopped

Instructions:

1. Preheat the oven to 400°F (200°C).
2. In a large bowl, combine the diced bell pepper, zucchini, yellow squash, and red onion. Drizzle with olive oil and sprinkle with dried oregano, salt, and pepper. Toss to coat the vegetables evenly.
3. Spread the vegetables in a single layer on a baking sheet and roast in the preheated oven for about 20-25 minutes, or until they are tender and slightly caramelized.
4. In a separate bowl, combine the cooked quinoa, roasted vegetables, lemon juice, and fresh parsley. Toss gently to combine.
5. Adjust the seasoning if needed. Serve the quinoa salad at room temperature or chilled.

Turkey Wrap with Lettuce and Avocado

Ingredients:

- 4 large whole wheat tortillas
- 8 slices of turkey breast
- 1 avocado, sliced
- 4 lettuce leaves
- 4 tablespoons hummus

Instructions:

1. Lay out the tortillas on a clean surface.
2. Spread 1 tablespoon of hummus on each tortilla.
3. Place 2 slices of turkey breast on each tortilla.
4. Top with avocado slices and a lettuce leaf.
5. Roll up the tortillas tightly, tucking in the sides as you go.
6. Cut each wrap in half diagonally. Serve immediately or wrap in foil for later.

Vegetable and Lentil Stew

Ingredients:

- 1 tablespoon olive oil

- 1 onion, diced
- 2 carrots, peeled and diced
- 2 celery stalks, diced
- 2 cloves of garlic, minced
- 1 cup green lentils, rinsed and drained
- 4 cups vegetable broth
- 1 can (14 ounces) diced tomatoes
- 1 teaspoon dried thyme
- Salt and pepper to taste
- Fresh parsley, chopped (for garnish)

Instructions:

1. Heat the olive oil in a large pot over medium heat. Add the onion, carrots, celery, and garlic. Sauté until the vegetables are tender.
2. Add the green lentils, vegetable broth, diced tomatoes, dried thyme, salt, and pepper. Stir well to combine.
3. Bring the stew to a boil, then reduce the heat to low and simmer for about 30-40 minutes, or until the lentils are cooked and tender.

4. Adjust the seasoning if needed. Serve hot, garnished with fresh parsley.

Greek Salad with Grilled Chicken

Ingredients:

- 2 chicken breasts
- 2 tablespoons olive oil
- 1 teaspoon dried oregano
- Salt and pepper to tast4 cups mixed salad greens
- 1 cucumber, diced
- 1 tomato, diced
- 1/2 red onion, thinly sliced
- 1/4 cup Kalamata olives
- 1/4 cup crumbled feta cheese
- Lemon wedges (for serving)

Instructions:

1. Preheat the grill to medium-high heat.
2. Brush the chicken breasts with olive oil and sprinkle with dried oregano, salt, and pepper.

3. Grill the chicken for about 6-8 minutes per side, or until cooked through and no longer pink in the center. Let the chicken rest for a few minutes before slicing.

4. In a large bowl, combine the mixed salad greens, cucumber, tomato, red onion, Kalamata olives, and crumbled feta cheese. Toss to combine.

5. Divide the salad onto plates and top with sliced grilled chicken. Serve with lemon wedges on the side for squeezing over the salad.

Tuna Salad Lettuce Wraps

Ingredients:

- 2 cans (5 ounces each) tuna, drained
- 1/4 cup mayonnaise
- 2 tablespoons Dijon mustard
- 2 celery stalks, diced
- 1/4 cup red onion, diced
- Salt and pepper to taste
- 8 large lettuce leaves

Instructions:

1. In a bowl, combine the tuna, mayonnaise, Dijon
    mustard, celery, red onion, salt, and pepper. Mix well
    to combine.
2. Lay out the lettuce leaves on a clean surface.
3. Spoon the tuna salad onto each lettuce leaf.
4. Roll up the lettuce leaves, tucking in the sides as you
    go.
5. Cut each wrap in half diagonally. Serve immediately
    or refrigerate until ready to eat.

Egg Salad Sandwich on Whole Grain Bread

Ingredients:

- 6 hard-boiled eggs, peeled and chopped
- 1/4 cup mayonnaise
- 1 tablespoon Dijon mustard
- 2 green onions, thinly sliced
- Salt and pepper to taste
- 8 slices whole grain bread
- Lettuce leaves (optional)

Instructions:

1. In a bowl, combine the chopped hard-boiled eggs, mayonnaise, Dijon mustard, green onions, salt, and pepper. Mix well to combine.
2. Lay out the slices of whole grain bread on a clean surface.
3. Spread a generous amount of the egg salad mixture onto 4 slices of bread.
4. Top with lettuce leaves if desired, then cover with the remaining 4 slices of bread.
5. Cut the sandwiches in half diagonally. Serve immediately or wrap in foil for later.

Roasted Butternut Squash Soup

Ingredients:

- 1 medium butternut squash, peeled, seeded, and cubed
- 1 onion, diced
- 2 carrots, peeled and diced
- 2 celery stalks, diced
- 2 cloves of garlic, minced
- 2 tablespoons olive oil
- 4 cups vegetable broth

- 1 teaspoon dried thyme
- Salt and pepper to taste
- 1/4 cup heavy cream (optional)
- Fresh parsley, chopped (for garnish)

Instructions:

1. Preheat the oven to 400°F (200°C).
2. Place the cubed butternut squash, diced onion, carrots, celery, and minced garlic on a baking sheet. Drizzle with olive oil and sprinkle with dried thyme, salt, and pepper. Toss to coat the vegetables evenly.
3. Roast the vegetables in the preheated oven for about 25-30 minutes, or until they are tender and slightly caramelized.
4. Transfer the roasted vegetables to a large pot. Add the vegetable broth and bring to a boil. Reduce the heat to low and simmer for about 10 minutes.
5. Using an immersion blender or regular blender, puree the soup until smooth and creamy.
6. Stir in the heavy cream if desired. Adjust the seasoning if needed.

7. Serve the roasted butternut squash soup hot, garnished with fresh parsley.

Quinoa Stuffed Bell Peppers

Ingredients:

- 4 bell peppers (any color), tops cut off and seeds removed
- 1 cup quinoa, cooked
- 1 cup black beans, rinsed and drained
- 1 cup corn kernels
- 1/2 cup diced tomatoes
- 1/4 cup red onion, diced
- 1/4 cup fresh cilantro, chopped
- 1 teaspoon ground cumin
- 1/2 teaspoon chili powder
- Salt and pepper to taste
- 1/2 cup shredded cheddar cheese (optional)

Instructions:

1. Preheat the oven to 375°F (190°C).
2. In a bowl, combine the cooked quinoa, black beans, corn kernels, diced tomatoes, red onion, cilantro,

ground cumin, chili powder, salt, and pepper. Mix well to combine.

3. Stuff each bell pepper with the quinoa mixture and place them in a baking dish.

4. If using cheese, sprinkle the shredded cheddar cheese over the stuffed bell peppers.

5. Cover the baking dish with foil and bake in the preheated oven for about 25-30 minutes, or until the bell peppers are tender and the filling is heated through.

6. Remove the foil and bake for an additional 5 minutes, or until the cheese is melted and bubbly (if using).

7. Serve the quinoa stuffed bell peppers hot, optionally garnished with additional cilantro.

Dinner Recipes

In this chapter, we will explore delicious and nutritious dinner recipes that are perfect for those following a low residue diet. These recipes offer a variety of flavors and ingredients to keep your taste buds satisfied while still being gentle on your digestive system. From tender baked chicken breast with creamy mashed potatoes to flavorful grilled shrimp with quinoa pilaf, these dishes are sure to become family favorites. So, let's dive into the recipes and discover new dinner options that are both wholesome and enjoyable.

Baked Chicken Breast with Mashed Potatoes

Ingredients:

- 4 boneless, skinless chicken breasts
- 2 tablespoons olive oil
- 1 teaspoon garlic powder
- 1 teaspoon paprika
- Salt and pepper to taste
- 4 medium-sized potatoes, peeled and quartered

- ¼ cup unsalted butter

- ½ cup low-fat milk

- Chopped fresh parsley for garnish

Instructions:

1. Preheat the oven to 400°F (200°C).

2. In a small bowl, mix together the olive oil, garlic powder, paprika, salt, and pepper.

3. Place the chicken breasts on a baking sheet lined with parchment paper. Brush the chicken breasts with the olive oil mixture on both sides.

4. Bake the chicken in the preheated oven for 25-30 minutes or until cooked through and no longer pink in the center.

5. While the chicken is baking, place the potatoes in a large pot of salted water. Bring to a boil and cook until tender, approximately 15-20 minutes.

6. Drain the potatoes and return them to the pot. Add the butter and milk to the pot and mash the potatoes until smooth and creamy. Season with salt and pepper to taste.

7. Serve the baked chicken breast with a generous scoop of mashed potatoes. Garnish with chopped fresh parsley.

Lemon Herb Grilled Shrimp with Quinoa Pilaf

Ingredients:

- 1 pound large shrimp, peeled and deveined
- Zest and juice of 1 lemon
- 2 tablespoons olive oil
- 2 cloves garlic, minced
- 1 tablespoon chopped fresh parsley
- 1 tablespoon chopped fresh basil
- Salt and pepper to taste
- 1 cup quinoa
- 2 cups low-sodium chicken or vegetable broth
- 1 small onion, finely chopped
- 1 carrot, finely chopped
- 1 celery stalk, finely chopped

Instructions:

1. In a large bowl, combine the shrimp, lemon zest, lemon juice, olive oil, minced garlic, parsley, basil, salt, and pepper. Toss until the shrimp is well coated. Let it marinate in the refrigerator for at least 30 minutes.

2. Preheat the grill to medium-high heat.

3. In a medium-sized saucepan, combine the quinoa and broth. Bring to a boil, then reduce the heat to low, cover, and simmer for 15-20 minutes or until the quinoa is tender and the liquid is absorbed.

4. Meanwhile, thread the marinated shrimp onto skewers.

5. Grill the shrimp skewers for 2-3 minutes per side or until the shrimp is opaque and cooked through.

6. In a separate pan, sauté the onion, carrot, and celery until they are tender.

7. Fluff the cooked quinoa with a fork and stir in the sautéed vegetables. Season with salt and pepper to taste.

8. Serve the grilled shrimp skewers over the quinoa pilaf.

Roasted Turkey Breast with Steamed Broccoli

Ingredients:

- 1 boneless turkey breast, approximately 2 pounds
- 2 tablespoons olive oil
- 1 teaspoon dried thyme
- 1 teaspoon dried rosemary
- Salt and pepper to taste
- 4 cups broccoli florets
- 1 tablespoon lemon juice

Instructions:

1. Preheat the oven to 375°F (190°C).
2. Rub the turkey breast with olive oil and sprinkle with dried thyme, dried rosemary, salt, and pepper.
3. Place the turkey breast on a baking sheet lined with parchment paper. Roast in the preheated oven for 1 to 1.5 hours, or until the internal temperature reaches 165°F (74°C).
4. While the turkey is roasting, steam the broccoli florets until tender, approximately 5-7 minutes.

5. Once the turkey is cooked, remove it from the oven and let it rest for 10 minutes before slicing.
6. Toss the steamed broccoli with lemon juice.
7. Slice the roasted turkey breast and serve with a side of steamed broccoli.

Baked Cod with Sweet Potato Mash

Ingredients:

- 4 cod fillets
- 2 tablespoons lemon juice
- 2 tablespoons olive oil
- 1 teaspoon dried dill
- Salt and pepper to taste
- 2 large sweet potatoes, peeled and cubed
- 2 tablespoons unsalted butter
- ¼ cup low-fat milk
- Chopped fresh parsley for garnish

Instructions:

1. Preheat the oven to 400°F (200°C).

2. Place the cod fillets in a baking dish. Drizzle with lemon juice and olive oil. Sprinkle with dried dill, salt, and pepper.

3. Bake the cod in the preheated oven for 12-15 minutes or until it flakes easily with a fork.

4. While the cod is baking, place the sweet potato cubes in a pot of salted water. Bring to a boil and cook until the sweet potatoes are tender, approximately 10-12 minutes.

5. Drain the sweet potatoes and return them to the pot. Add the butter and milk to the pot and mash the sweet potatoes until smooth and creamy. Season with salt and pepper to taste.

6. Serve the baked cod fillets with a scoop of sweet potato mash. Garnish with chopped fresh parsley.

Vegetable Stir-Fry with Brown Rice

Ingredients:

- 2 cups cooked brown rice
- 2 tablespoons low-sodium soy sauce
- 1 tablespoon sesame oil 1 tablespoon olive oil
- 1 small onion, thinly sliced

- 2 cloves garlic, minced
- 1 cup sliced mushrooms
- 1 cup sliced bell peppers (assorted colors)
- 1 cup sliced zucchini
- 1 cup broccoli florets
- 1 cup snap peas
- Salt and pepper to taste
- Chopped green onions for garnish

Instructions:

1. Heat the sesame oil and olive oil in a large skillet or wok over medium-high heat.
2. Add the onion and garlic to the skillet and sauté until fragrant and slightly softened.
3. Add the mushrooms, bell peppers, zucchini, broccoli, and snap peas to the skillet. Stir-fry for 5-7 minutes or until the vegetables are tender-crisp.
4. In a small bowl, whisk together the soy sauce and a dash of sesame oil. Pour the sauce over the vegetables and toss to coat evenly. Season with salt and pepper to taste.

5. Add the cooked brown rice to the skillet and stir-fry for an additional 2-3 minutes, until heated through.

6. Serve the vegetable stir-fry over a bed of brown rice. Garnish with chopped green onions.

Beef and Vegetable Skewers with Couscous

Ingredients:

- 1 pound beef sirloin, cut into 1-inch cubes
- 1 red bell pepper, cut into chunks
- 1 green bell pepper, cut into chunks
- 1 red onion, cut into chunks
- 8 cherry tomatoes
- 2 tablespoons olive oil
- 2 tablespoons balsamic vinegar
- 2 cloves garlic, minced
- 1 teaspoon dried oregano
- Salt and pepper to taste
- 1 cup couscous
- 1¼ cups low-sodium beef or vegetable broth
- Chopped fresh parsley for garnish

Instructions:

1. Preheat the grill or broiler to medium-high heat.

2. Thread the beef cubes, bell peppers, red onion, and cherry tomatoes onto skewers, alternating the ingredients.

3. In a small bowl, whisk together the olive oil, balsamic vinegar, minced garlic, dried oregano, salt, and pepper.

4. Brush the skewers with the marinade, reserving some for basting during cooking.

5. Grill or broil the skewers for 10-12 minutes, turning occasionally and basting with the reserved marinade, until the beef is cooked to your desired doneness and the vegetables are tender.

6. While the skewers are cooking, prepare the couscous according to the package instructions, using the low-sodium beef or vegetable broth instead of water.

7. Fluff the cooked couscous with a fork and serve alongside the beef and vegetable skewers. Garnish with chopped fresh parsley.

Zucchini Noodles with Tomato Sauce

Ingredients:

- 4 medium zucchini
- 2 tablespoons olive oil
- 2 cloves garlic, minced
- 1 can (14 ounces) crushed tomatoes
- 1 teaspoon dried basil
- 1 teaspoon dried oregano
- Salt and pepper to taste
- Grated Parmesan cheese for garnish
- Fresh basil leaves for garnish

Instructions:

1. Using a spiralizer or vegetable peeler, cut the zucchini into thin noodle-like strips.
2. Heat the olive oil in a large skillet over medium heat. Add the minced garlic and sauté for 1 minute, until fragrant.
3. Add the crushed tomatoes, dried basil, dried oregano, salt, and pepper to the skillet. Simmer for 10-15 minutes to allow the flavors to meld together.

4. In a separate pan, sauté the zucchini noodles in a little olive oil for 2-3 minutes, or until tender.

5. Divide the zucchini noodles into serving bowls and top with the tomato sauce.

6. Garnish with grated Parmesan cheese and fresh basil leaves before serving.

Grilled Pork Tenderloin with Roasted Vegetables

Ingredients:

- 1 pound pork tenderloin
- 2 tablespoons olive oil
- 2 cloves garlic, minced
- 1 teaspoon dried thyme
- Salt and pepper to taste
- 2 cups mixed vegetables (such as carrots, bell peppers, and Brussels sprouts), cut into bite-sized pieces
- 1 tablespoon balsamic vinegar

Instructions:

1. Preheat the grill to medium-high heat.

2. In a small bowl, combine the olive oil, minced garlic, dried thyme, salt, and pepper. Rub the mixture over the pork tenderloin to coat evenly.

3. Grill the pork tenderloin for 15-20 minutes, turning occasionally, until the internal temperature reaches 145°F (63°C).

4. While the pork is grilling, preheat the oven to 400°F (200°C).

5. Toss the mixed vegetables with olive oil, salt, and pepper. Spread them out in a single layer on a baking sheet and roast in the preheated oven for 15-20 minutes, or until tender and lightly browned.

6. Remove the pork tenderloin from the grill and let it rest for 5 minutes before slicing.

7. Drizzle the roasted vegetables with balsamic vinegar and serve alongside the sliced pork tenderloin.

Stuffed Portobello Mushrooms with Quinoa

Ingredients:

- 4 large Portobello mushrooms
- 2 tablespoons olive oil

- 1 small onion, finely chopped
- 2 cloves garlic, minced
- 1 cup cooked quinoa
- 1 cup chopped spinach
- ½ cup crumbled feta cheese
- ¼ cup chopped sun-dried tomatoes
- Salt and pepper to taste
- Fresh parsley for garnish

Instructions:

1. Preheat the oven to 375°F (190°C).
2. Remove the stems from the Portobello mushrooms and gently scrape out the gills with a spoon. Brush the mushrooms with olive oil on both sides and place them on a baking sheet lined with parchment paper.
3. In a skillet, heat the olive oil over medium heat. Add the chopped onion and minced garlic and sauté until softened and fragrant.
4. Add the cooked quinoa, chopped spinach, crumbled feta cheese, and chopped sun-dried tomatoes to the skillet. Stir well to combine. Season with salt and pepper to taste.

5. Spoon the quinoa mixture into the Portobello mushrooms, pressing it down gently.

6. Bake the stuffed mushrooms in the preheated oven for 20-25 minutes, or until the mushrooms are tender and the filling is heated through.

7. Garnish with fresh parsley before serving.

Lentil and Vegetable Curry

Ingredients:

- 1 cup dried lentils, rinsed and drained
- 2 tablespoons olive oil
- 1 small onion, finely chopped
- 2 cloves garlic, minced
- 1 tablespoon curry powder
- 1 teaspoon ground cumin
- 1 teaspoon ground coriander
- ½ teaspoon turmeric
- ½ teaspoon paprika
- 2 cups chopped mixed vegetables (such as carrots, bell peppers, and cauliflower)
- 1 can (14 ounces) coconut milk
- 1 cup low-sodium vegetable broth

- Salt and pepper to taste
- Chopped fresh cilantro for garnish

Instructions:

1. Cook the lentils according to the package instructions. Drain and set aside.
2. In a large skillet, heat the olive oil over medium heat. Add the chopped onion and minced garlic and sauté until softened and fragrant.
3. Add the curry powder, ground cumin, ground coriander, turmeric, and paprika to the skillet. Stir well to coat the onions and garlic with the spices.
4. Add the chopped mixed vegetables to the skillet and sauté for 5-7 minutes, or until they are slightly tender.
5. Stir in the cooked lentils, coconut milk, and vegetable broth. Bring to a simmer and cook for 10-15 minutes to allow the flavors to meld together. Season with salt and pepper to taste.
6. Serve the lentil and vegetable curry over cooked rice or quinoa. Garnish with chopped fresh cilantro.

Snacks and Appetizers

In this chapter, you'll discover a variety of delightful snacks and appetizers that are not only delicious but also suitable for a low residue diet. These recipes incorporate wholesome ingredients and are easy to prepare. Get ready to tantalize your taste buds with these flavorful treats!

Rice Cakes with Hummus and Cucumber Slices

Ingredients:

- 4 rice cakes
- 1/2 cup hummus
- 1 cucumber, thinly sliced

Instructions:

1. Spread a generous amount of hummus on each rice cake.
2. Top the hummus with a few slices of cucumber.
3. Serve immediately and enjoy the crunchy and refreshing combination of flavors.

Greek Yogurt with Fresh Berries

Ingredients:

- 1 cup Greek yogurt
- 1/2 cup fresh berries (such as strawberries, blueberries, or raspberries)
- 1 tablespoon honey (optional)

Instructions:

1. In a serving bowl or glass, spoon the Greek yogurt.
2. Scatter the fresh berries on top of the yogurt.
3. Drizzle honey over the berries, if desired, for added sweetness.
4. Mix everything gently to combine the flavors.
5. Enjoy this nutritious and delicious snack packed with protein and antioxidants.

Carrot and Celery Sticks with Almond Butter

Ingredients:

- 2 carrots, peeled and cut into sticks
- 2 celery stalks, cut into sticks
- 1/4 cup almond butter

Instructions:

1. Arrange the carrot and celery sticks on a plate.

2. Place the almond butter in a small bowl for dipping.

3. Dip the carrot and celery sticks into the almond butter and savor the crunchy texture and nutty flavor.

4. This snack is rich in vitamins, fiber, and healthy fats.

Baked Kale Chips

Ingredients:

- 1 bunch kale, washed and dried
- 1 tablespoon olive oil
- Salt and pepper to taste

Instructions:

1. Preheat the oven to 350°F (175°C) and line a baking sheet with parchment paper.

2. Remove the tough stems from the kale leaves and tear them into bite-sized pieces.

3. In a bowl, toss the kale with olive oil, salt, and pepper until evenly coated.

4. Arrange the kale pieces in a single layer on the prepared baking sheet.

5. Bake for about 10-15 minutes until the edges are crispy but not burnt.

6. Let the kale chips cool for a few minutes before enjoying their crispy and flavorful goodness.

Cucumber and Tomato Salad

Ingredients:

- 1 cucumber, diced
- 1 cup cherry tomatoes, halved
- 2 tablespoons red onion, finely chopped
- 2 tablespoons fresh parsley, chopped
- 1 tablespoon lemon juice
- 1 tablespoon olive oil
- Salt and pepper to taste

Instructions:

1. In a bowl, combine the cucumber, cherry tomatoes, red onion, and parsley.

2. In a separate small bowl, whisk together lemon juice, olive oil, salt, and pepper to make the dressing.

3. Pour the dressing over the cucumber and tomato mixture and toss gently to coat.

4. Refrigerate the salad for at least 30 minutes to allow
    the flavors to meld.

5. Serve chilled as a refreshing and vibrant snack.

Mini Quiche Cups

Ingredients:

- 6 large eggs
- 1/4 cup milk
- 1/2 cup shredded cheese (such as cheddar or Swiss)
- 1/4 cup diced vegetables (such as bell peppers, spinach, or mushrooms)
- Salt and pepper to taste

Instructions:

1. Preheat the oven to 375°F (190°C) and grease a muffin tin.

2. In a bowl, whisk together the eggs, milk, salt, and pepper.

3. Divide the diced vegetables and shredded cheese evenly among the muffin cups.

4. Pour the egg mixture over the vegetables and cheese, filling each cup about 3/4 full.

5. Bake for 20-25 minutes or until the quiche cups are puffed and set in the center.

6. Allow them to cool slightly before removing from the muffin tin.

7. Serve these mini quiche cups as a tasty and protein-packed appetizer or snack.

Spinach and Artichoke Dip with Whole Grain Crackers

Ingredients:

- 1 cup frozen spinach, thawed and squeezed dry
- 1 cup canned artichoke hearts, drained and chopped
- 1/2 cup Greek yogurt
- 1/2 cup mayonnaise
- 1/4 cup grated Parmesan cheese
- 1/4 cup shredded mozzarella cheese
- 1 clove garlic, minced
- Salt and pepper to taste
- Whole grain crackers for serving

Instructions:

1. Preheat the oven to 375°F (190°C).

2. In a mixing bowl, combine the spinach, artichoke hearts, Greek yogurt, mayonnaise, Parmesan cheese, mozzarella cheese, garlic, salt, and pepper.

3. Mix well until all the ingredients are thoroughly combined.

4. Transfer the mixture to a baking dish and spread it evenly.

5. Bake for 20-25 minutes or until the top is golden and bubbly.

6. Remove from the oven and let it cool slightly before serving with whole grain crackers.

7. Enjoy this creamy and flavorful dip as a crowd-pleasing appetizer.

Apple Slices with Peanut Butter

Ingredients:

- 2 apples, cored and sliced
- 1/4 cup peanut butter
- Optional toppings: chopped nuts, raisins, or honey

Instructions:

1. Arrange the apple slices on a plate.

2. Place the peanut butter in a small bowl for dipping.

3. Dip the apple slices into the peanut butter and add optional toppings for added flavor and texture.

4. Indulge in this simple and satisfying snack that combines the natural sweetness of apples with the richness of peanut butter.

Roasted Chickpeas

Ingredients:

- 1 can chickpeas (15 ounces), drained and rinsed
- 1 tablespoon olive oil
- 1 teaspoon ground cumin
- 1/2 teaspoon paprika
- 1/2 teaspoon garlic powder
- Salt to taste

Instructions:

1. Preheat the oven to 400°F (200°C) and line a baking sheet with parchment paper.

2. In a bowl, toss the chickpeas with olive oil, cumin, paprika, garlic powder, and salt until well coated.

3. Spread the seasoned chickpeas in a single layer on the prepared baking sheet.

4. Roast for about 20-25 minutes, stirring once or twice, until the chickpeas are crispy and golden brown.

5. Allow them to cool slightly before munching on these crunchy and protein-packed roasted chickpeas.

Veggie Sushi Rolls

Ingredients:

- 4 nori seaweed sheets
- 2 cups cooked sushi rice
- 1/2 cucumber, julienned
- 1 carrot, julienned
- 1/2 avocado, thinly sliced
- Soy sauce and wasabi for serving

Instructions:

1. Place a nori seaweed sheet on a bamboo sushi mat or a clean surface.

2. Spread an even layer of sushi rice on the nori sheet, leaving about 1 inch at the top empty.

3. Arrange the cucumber, carrot, and avocado slices horizontally on the rice.

4. Roll the sushi tightly using the bamboo mat or your hands, starting from the bottom edge.

5. Wet the top edge of the nori sheet with water to seal the roll.

6. Repeat the process with the remaining nori sheets and fillings.

7. Slice each sushi roll into bite-sized pieces using a sharp knife.

8. Serve the veggie sushi rolls with soy sauce and wasabi for dipping.

9. Enjoy these homemade sushi rolls as a flavorful and healthy snack or appetizer.

Desserts

Indulge in these delectable dessert recipes that are not only delicious but also suitable for a low residue diet. Each recipe offers a delightful treat while prioritizing gentle digestion. Whether you're craving fruity, chocolaty, or creamy flavors, this chapter has a dessert option to satisfy your taste buds. From frozen delights to comforting puddings, these desserts will make your low residue diet a little more enjoyable.

Banana Ice Cream with Almond Butter Drizzle

Ingredients:

- 4 ripe bananas
- ¼ cup almond butter
- 2 tablespoons honey
- ½ teaspoon vanilla extract
- Optional toppings: chopped nuts, shredded coconut, chocolate chips

Instructions:

1. Peel the bananas and cut them into small chunks. Place the banana chunks in a freezer bag and freeze them for at least 2 hours or until completely frozen.

2. Once the bananas are frozen, transfer them to a blender or food processor.

3. Add almond butter, honey, and vanilla extract to the blender.

4. Blend the mixture until smooth and creamy, scraping down the sides of the blender as needed.

5. Transfer the banana ice cream to a container and freeze for an additional 1-2 hours to firm up.

6. Serve the banana ice cream in bowls or cones and drizzle with almond butter. Add optional toppings if desired.

7. Enjoy the creamy and delicious banana ice cream with almond butter drizzle!

Baked Apples with Cinnamon and Walnuts

Ingredients:

- 4 apples (Honeycrisp, Granny Smith, or any other baking apple)

- ¼ cup chopped walnuts

- 2 tablespoons honey

- 1 teaspoon ground cinnamon

- 1 tablespoon butter, melted

Instructions:

1. Preheat your oven to 350°F (175°C).

2. Wash the apples thoroughly and core them, leaving the bottoms intact.

3. In a small bowl, combine the chopped walnuts, honey, cinnamon, and melted butter.

4. Stuff the mixture into the center of each apple, filling it generously.

5. Place the stuffed apples in a baking dish and bake for 30-35 minutes or until the apples are tender.

6. Remove from the oven and let them cool for a few minutes.

7. Serve the baked apples warm, optionally topped with a dollop of Greek yogurt or a scoop of vanilla ice cream.

Mixed Berry Smoothie Bowl

Ingredients:

- 1 cup frozen mixed berries (strawberries, blueberries, raspberries)
- 1 ripe banana
- ½ cup plain Greek yogurt
- ¼ cup almond milk (or any other milk of your choice)
- Toppings: granola, sliced fresh berries, chia seeds, shredded coconut

Instructions:

1. In a blender, combine the frozen mixed berries, ripe banana, Greek yogurt, and almond milk.
2. Blend until smooth and creamy, adding more almond milk if needed to reach the desired consistency.
3. Pour the smoothie into a bowl.
4. Top with your favorite toppings such as granola, sliced fresh berries, chia seeds, and shredded coconut.
5. Enjoy the refreshing and nutritious mixed berry smoothie bowl as a satisfying breakfast or snack.

Chocolate Avocado Pudding

Ingredients:

- 2 ripe avocados
- ¼ cup unsweetened cocoa powder
- ¼ cup honey or maple syrup
- ½ teaspoon vanilla extract
- Pinch of salt
- Optional toppings: fresh berries, chopped nuts, shredded coconut

Instructions:

1. Cut the avocados in half, remove the pits, and scoop out the flesh into a blender or food processor.
2. Add the cocoa powder, honey or maple syrup, vanilla extract, and salt to the blender.
3. Blend until smooth and creamy, scraping down the sides of the blender as needed.
4. Transfer the pudding to serving bowls or glasses.
5. Chill in the refrigerator for at least 1 hour to allow the flavors to meld.
6. Garnish with fresh berries, chopped nuts, or shredded coconut if desired.

7. Indulge in the rich and velvety chocolate avocado pudding, a healthier alternative to traditional pudding recipes.

Yogurt Parfait with Granola and Fresh Fruit

Ingredients:

- 1 cup Greek yogurt
- ¼ cup granola
- ½ cup fresh mixed berries (strawberries, blueberries, raspberries)
- 2 tablespoons honey

Instructions:

1. In a glass or a jar, layer the Greek yogurt, granola, and fresh mixed berries.
2. Drizzle honey over the top.
3. Repeat the layers until all the ingredients are used, ending with a dollop of Greek yogurt and a sprinkle of granola.

4. Serve immediately and enjoy the delightful combination of creamy yogurt, crunchy granola, and sweet fresh fruit.

Chia Seed Chocolate Pudding

Ingredients:

- ¼ cup chia seeds
- 1 cup almond milk (or any other milk of your choice)
- 2 tablespoons unsweetened cocoa powder
- 2 tablespoons honey or maple syrup
- ½ teaspoon vanilla extract
- Optional toppings: sliced bananas, berries, chopped nuts

Instructions:

1. In a bowl, combine the chia seeds, almond milk, cocoa powder, honey or maple syrup, and vanilla extract.
2. Whisk well to ensure the cocoa powder is fully incorporated.
3. Let the mixture sit for 5 minutes, then whisk again to break up any clumps.

4. Cover the bowl and refrigerate for at least 2 hours or overnight, allowing the chia seeds to absorb the liquid and create a pudding-like consistency.

5. Stir the pudding before serving and add optional toppings such as sliced bananas, berries, or chopped nuts.

6. Enjoy the nutritious and satisfying chia seed chocolate pudding as a guilt-free dessert or snack.

Coconut Macaroons

Ingredients:

- 2 cups shredded coconut (unsweetened)
- ⅔ cup sweetened condensed milk
- 2 egg whites
- 1 teaspoon vanilla extract
- Pinch of salt

Instructions:

- Preheat your oven to 325°F (165°C) and line a baking sheet with parchment paper.
- In a bowl, combine the shredded coconut, sweetened condensed milk, vanilla extract, and salt. Mix well.

- In a separate bowl, beat the egg whites until stiff peaks form.

- Gently fold the beaten egg whites into the coconut mixture until fully combined.

- Drop rounded tablespoonfuls of the mixture onto the prepared baking sheet, spacing them apart.

- Bake for 15-18 minutes or until the macaroons turn golden brown on the edges.

- Remove from the oven and let them cool completely before serving.

- Enjoy the sweet and chewy coconut macaroons as a delightful treat with a hint of tropical flavor.

Grilled Pineapple with Honey and Cinnamon

Ingredients:

- 1 ripe pineapple, peeled and cored
- 2 tablespoons honey
- ½ teaspoon ground cinnamon
- Optional toppings: vanilla ice cream, chopped mint leaves

Instructions:

1. Preheat your grill or grill pan over medium heat.
2. Slice the pineapple into rings or wedges, about ½ inch thick.
3. In a small bowl, combine the honey and ground cinnamon.
4. Brush the pineapple slices with the honey-cinnamon mixture, coating both sides.
5. Grill the pineapple slices for 2-3 minutes per side, until grill marks appear and the pineapple is heated through.
6. Remove from the grill and transfer to a serving plate.
7. Serve the grilled pineapple slices as is or with a scoop of vanilla ice cream and a sprinkle of chopped mint leaves for added freshness.

Strawberry Shortcake Cups

Ingredients:

- 1 cup all-purpose flou
- ¼ cup granulated sugar
- 1 teaspoon baking powder
- ¼ teaspoon salt

- ½ cup unsalted butter, cold and cut into small pieces
- ¼ cup milk
- 1 teaspoon vanilla extract
- 2 cups fresh strawberries, hulled and sliced
- Whipped cream or Greek yogurt, for serving

Instructions:

1. Preheat your oven to 375°F (190°C) and line a baking sheet with parchment paper.
2. In a bowl, whisk together the flour, granulated sugar, baking powder, and salt.
3. Add the cold butter pieces to the dry ingredients and use a pastry cutter or your fingertips to cut the butter into the flour mixture until it resembles coarse crumbs.
4. In a separate bowl, combine the milk and vanilla extract.
5. Gradually pour the milk mixture into the flour mixture, stirring until the dough comes together.
6. Turn the dough out onto a lightly floured surface and knead it a few times until it forms a smooth ball.

7. Roll out the dough to a ¼-inch thickness and cut it into small rounds or squares using a cookie cutter or a sharp knife.

8. Place the shortcake cups onto the prepared baking sheet and bake for 12-15 minutes or until golden brown.

9. Remove from the oven and let them cool completely.

10. To assemble the strawberry shortcake cups, spoon a generous amount of sliced strawberries onto each cup and top with whipped cream or Greek yogurt.

11. Serve the delightful strawberry shortcake cups as a classic and charming dessert.

Rice Pudding with Cinnamon and Raisins

Ingredients:

- ½ cup white rice
- 2 cups whole milk
- ¼ cup granulated sugar
- ½ teaspoon ground cinnamon
- ¼ cup raisins
- 1 teaspoon vanilla extract

Instructions:

1. In a medium-sized saucepan, combine the white rice, whole milk, granulated sugar, ground cinnamon, and raisins.

2. Bring the mixture to a boil over medium heat, then reduce the heat to low and simmer, stirring occasionally, for about 25-30 minutes or until the rice is tender and the mixture thickens.

3. Remove the saucepan from the heat and stir in the vanilla extract.

4. Let the rice pudding cool for a few minutes before serving.

5. Serve the warm or chilled rice pudding in bowls, optionally sprinkled with additional cinnamon on top.

6. Enjoy the comforting and creamy rice pudding with hints of cinnamon and sweet raisins.

Smoothies

Smoothies are not only delicious but also a great way to incorporate a variety of nutritious ingredients into your diet. In this chapter, we will explore ten different smoothie recipes that are not only tasty but also packed with vitamins, minerals, and antioxidants. Whether you're looking for a refreshing breakfast option or a satisfying afternoon snack, these smoothies are sure to please your taste buds and provide a healthy boost to your day.

Berry Blast Smoothie

Ingredients:

- 1 cup mixed berries (strawberries, blueberries, raspberries)
- 1 ripe banana
- 1/2 cup plain Greek yogurt
- 1/2 cup almond milk
- 1 tablespoon honey
- Ice cubes (optional)

Instructions:

1. Wash the berries and remove any stems.

2. Peel the banana and break it into chunks.

3. Place the berries, banana, Greek yogurt, almond milk, and honey in a blender.

4. Blend on high speed until smooth and creamy.

5. If desired, add a few ice cubes and blend again until well combined.

6. Pour into a glass and enjoy this delightful berry blast smoothie.

Green Detox Smoothie

Ingredients:

- 1 cup fresh spinach leaves

- 1/2 cucumber, peeled and chopped

- 1/2 green apple, cored and chopped

- 1/2 ripe avocado

- 1 tablespoon fresh lemon juice

- 1 cup coconut water

- Ice cubes (optional)

Instructions:

1. Rinse the spinach leaves thoroughly.

2. Peel and chop the cucumber and green apple.

3. Cut the avocado in half, remove the pit, and scoop out the flesh.

4. Place the spinach, cucumber, green apple, avocado, lemon juice, and coconut water in a blender.

5. Blend on high speed until smooth and creamy.

6. Add a few ice cubes if desired and blend again until well mixed.

7. Pour into a glass and enjoy this refreshing green detox smoothie.

Tropical Paradise Smoothie

Ingredients:

- 1/2 cup pineapple chunks
- 1/2 cup mango chunks
- 1/2 ripe banana
- 1/2 cup coconut milk
- 1/2 cup orange juice
- 1 tablespoon shredded coconut (optional)
- Ice cubes (optional)

Instructions:

1. Peel and chop the pineapple, mango, and banana.

2. Place the pineapple, mango, banana, coconut milk, orange juice, and shredded coconut (if using) in a blender.

3. Blend on high speed until smooth and creamy.

4. Add a few ice cubes if desired and blend again until well combined.

5. Pour into a glass, and imagine yourself in a tropical paradise as you sip on this delicious smoothie.

Peanut Butter Banana Smoothie

Ingredients:

- 1 ripe banana
- 2 tablespoons peanut butter
- 1 cup almond milk
- 1 tablespoon honey
- 1/2 teaspoon vanilla extract
- Ice cubes (optional)

Instructions:

1. Peel the banana and break it into chunks.

2. Place the banana, peanut butter, almond milk, honey, and vanilla extract in a blender.

3. Blend on high speed until smooth and creamy.

4. Add a few ice cubes if desired and blend again until well mixed.

5. Pour into a glass and indulge in the heavenly combination of peanut butter and banana in this smoothie.

Chocolate Almond Smoothie

Ingredients:

- 1 cup almond milk
- 1 ripe banana
- 2 tablespoons cocoa powder
- 1 tablespoon almond butter
- 1 tablespoon honey
- Ice cubes (optional)

Instructions:

1. Place the almond milk, banana, cocoa powder, almond butter, and honey in a blender.

2. Blend on high speed until smooth and creamy.

3. If desired, add a few ice cubes and blend again until well combined.

4. Pour into a glass and savor the rich and chocolatey goodness of this almond smoothie.

Mango Lassi Smoothie

Ingredients:

- 1 cup chopped mango
- 1/2 cup plain Greek yogurt
- 1/2 cup almond milk
- 1 tablespoon honey
- 1/4 teaspoon cardamom powder
- Ice cubes (optional)

Instructions:

1. Peel and chop the mango.
2. Place the chopped mango, Greek yogurt, almond milk, honey, and cardamom powder in a blender.
3. Blend on high speed until smooth and creamy.
4. Add a few ice cubes if desired and blend again until well mixed.

5. Pour into a glass and enjoy this refreshing and exotic mango lassi smoothie.

Spinach and Pineapple Smoothie

Ingredients:

- 1 cup fresh spinach leaves
- 1/2 cup pineapple chunks
- 1/2 ripe banana
- 1/2 cup coconut water
- 1 tablespoon fresh lime juice
- Ice cubes (optional)

Instructions:

1. Rinse the spinach leaves thoroughly.
2. Peel and chop the pineapple and banana.
3. Place the spinach, pineapple, banana, coconut water, and lime juice in a blender.
4. Blend on high speed until smooth and creamy.
5. Add a few ice cubes if desired and blend again until well combined.
6. Pour into a glass and enjoy this vibrant and nutritious spinach and pineapple smoothie.

Blueberry Coconut Smoothie

Ingredients:

- 1 cup blueberries
- 1/2 cup coconut milk
- 1/2 cup plain Greek yogurt
- 1 tablespoon honey
- 1/2 teaspoon vanilla extract
- Ice cubes (optional)

Instructions:

1. Wash the blueberries and remove any stems.
2. Place the blueberries, coconut milk, Greek yogurt, honey, and vanilla extract in a blender.
3. Blend on high speed until smooth and creamy.
4. Add a few ice cubes if desired and blend again until well mixed.
5. Pour into a glass and relish the delightful combination of blueberries and coconut in this smoothie.

Raspberry Vanilla Smoothie

Ingredients:

- 1 cup raspberries
- 1 cup almond milk
- 1/2 cup plain Greek yogurt
- 1 tablespoon honey
- 1/2 teaspoon vanilla extract
- Ice cubes (optional)

Instructions:

1. Wash the raspberries thoroughly.
2. Place the raspberries, almond milk, Greek yogurt, honey, and vanilla extract in a blender.
3. Blend on high speed until smooth and creamy.
4. Add a few ice cubes if desired and blend again until well combined.
5. Pour into a glass and savor the delicate flavors of raspberry and vanilla in this smoothie.

Peach and Ginger Smoothie

Ingredients:

- 1 ripe peach, pitted and chopped

- 1/2 cup almond milk

- 1/2 cup plain Greek yogurt

- 1 tablespoon honey

- 1 teaspoon grated ginger

- Ice cubes (optional)

Instructions:

1. Peel, pit, and chop the peach.

2. Place the chopped peach, almond milk, Greek yogurt, honey, and grated ginger in a blender.

3. Blend on high speed until smooth and creamy.

4. Add a few ice cubes if desired and blend again until well mixed.

5. Pour into a glass and enjoy the delightful combination of peach and ginger in this smoothie.

CONCLUSION

As we bring our journey through the Low Residue Diet Cookbook to a close. Throughout this cookbook, we have explored the principles, benefits, and recipes of a low residue diet. Now, let us reflect on the key takeaways and offer some concluding thoughts.

The low residue diet is a specialized eating plan designed to reduce the amount of fiber and undigested material in the digestive system. It is commonly prescribed for individuals with certain medical conditions, such as inflammatory bowel disease, diverticulitis, or after certain surgeries. By following a low residue diet, individuals can minimize bowel movements, decrease inflammation, and alleviate discomfort in the gastrointestinal tract.

Throughout this cookbook, we have provided a variety of delicious and nutritious recipes that adhere to the principles of a low residue diet. From breakfast to dinner, snacks to desserts, we have strived to offer a diverse range of options to suit different tastes and preferences. By incorporating these recipes into your daily routine, you can enjoy flavorful meals while adhering to the dietary guidelines of a low residue diet.

We began our journey with an introduction to the low residue diet, explaining its purpose and the benefits it offers. We discussed the importance of carefully selecting foods that are low in fiber, such as lean proteins, cooked fruits and vegetables, and refined grains. We also provided tips for success on the low residue diet, including the need for proper meal planning, staying hydrated, and consulting with a healthcare professional.

In subsequent chapters, we dived into specific meal categories, offering a collection of delectable recipes. Whether you were seeking a hearty breakfast to start your day, a satisfying lunch to keep you energized, a flavorful dinner to end your day on a high note, or a tempting snack or dessert to indulge in, we had you covered. We made sure to incorporate a range of ingredients and flavors to cater to different dietary preferences.

In addition to the main meal categories, we recognized the importance of snacks and appetizers in our daily lives. To satisfy those midday cravings or to enjoy a light bite between meals, we shared a selection of easy-to-prepare snacks and appetizers. From crispy kale chips to creamy hummus with fresh vegetables, these recipes provided a balance of nutrition and taste.

Furthermore, we acknowledged the importance of desserts in our culinary experiences. We presented a collection of delectable desserts that adhered to the guidelines of a low residue diet. From guilt-free fruit-based treats to creamy indulgences, these desserts allowed you to satisfy your sweet tooth while maintaining your dietary goals.

For those who prefer a refreshing and nutritious option, we dedicated a chapter solely to smoothies. These blended concoctions offered a convenient and delicious way to incorporate essential nutrients into your diet. From vibrant berry blends to creamy tropical delights, these smoothie recipes provided a refreshing break from traditional meals.

As we conclude this cookbook, it is important to remember that the low residue diet is not a one-size-fits-all approach. It is always advisable to consult with a healthcare professional or a registered dietitian before embarking on any significant dietary changes. They can provide personalized guidance based on your specific needs and health condition.

We hope that this cookbook has served as a valuable resource for individuals seeking to embrace a low residue diet. By offering a wide range of recipes and meal ideas, we aimed to make the dietary transition as seamless and enjoyable as possible. Remember to listen to your body,